Pain Management TA-DAs

Self Care Natural Techniques

PAIN MANAGEMENT TA-DAS

Self Care Natural Techniques

Julie E Spencer

Pain Management TA-DAs

Copyright © 2017 by Julie E Spencer

All rights reserved.

Published by Julie E Spencer

livinghands.net

Publishing Coaching: Erica and Lewis Rutherford, Jr.

Publishing and Marketing: CreateSpace.com

Photography by Bill Spencer

ISBN: 13:978-1545553862

ISBN: 10:1545553866

CONTENTS

DEDICATION	vi
ACKNOWLEDGEMENT	vii
INTRODUCTION	viii
TIPS AND TOOLS	ix
CHAPTER 1 TYPES OF PAIN	1
CHAPTER 2 TYPES OF PAIN MANAGEMENT	5
CHAPTER 3 TA-DAs	19
• LOWER BACK	26
• SHOULDERS	32
• DIGESTIVE	38
• BREATHING	39
• TMJ	43
• HEADACHES/MIGRAINES	48
• FEET	53
• HAND AND WRIST	57
CHAPTER 4 ESSENTIAL OILS	63
CHAPTER 5 HEALTHY FOODS/HERBS	76
CHAPTER 6 HERBAL SUPPLEMENTS	84
ABOUT AUTHOR	87
REFERENCES	88

DEDICATION

I dedicate this book to my Mom and Dad, Ruth "Naomi" and Bill Spencer, for all your support and encouragement in building me up, to know that I can go after my dreams, even with dyslexia and vision complications. Although you are with the Lord, you are always in my thoughts and heart.

ACKNOWLEDGEMENTS

For most, I thank our LORD for providing me the knowledge and GIFT to share these techniques, and the courage to write this book.

Thank you to all my friends and family who supported me while I dare to go after my dreams.

Thank you to Dr Shawn M. Pala, Chiropractic Physician of Pala Chiropractic and Sara Rodefeld, Certified Acupuncturist for sharing your knowledge.

Thank you to Bill Spencer, for his awesome use of the camera. For a picture is worth a thousand words.

Thank you to all of you for wanting to find a more natural way to manage your pain.

INTRODUCTION

Pain Management TA-DAs was written to help others who suffer from acute or chronic pain to have natural options to manage their pain. In this book I share several of the techniques that I do on myself to help with daily chronic pain from whiplash scar tissue, degenerative discs, osteoporosis, the permanent effects of advanced mold poisoning, fibromyalgia and scoliosis.

I have included some other natural treatments I have found to help as well. Such as, chiropractic treatment, herbal supplements, nutritional changes and essential oils.

Although there are numerous ways to manage pain, I am praying that some of these TA-DAs would shed some light on other options and some relief so you can live a more comfortable and active life.

> **All these techniques should be cleared with your physician before giving them a try.**

Are you ready to see how living with less pain can feel like? Let's go!

TIPS AND TOOLS

TIPS

- **SEEK MEDICAL EVALUATION BEFORE TRYING ANY OF THE TA-DAS OR ESSENTIAL OIL/SUPPLEMENTS to ensure there are no serious medical issues.** Get into your healthcare provider as soon as you can for maximum relief such as a medical doctor, massage therapist, chiropractor, acupuncturist, or physical therapist.
- When doing the TA-DAs they become more effective when breathing slowly and steady.
- Drink plenty of water – your body can only handle 8oz of water an hour. Drink less and more often.
- When doing the TA-DAs, if you find the muscles are not relaxing, lighten up on the pressure.

TOOLS

Here are some of the tools I use that may allow for ease when doing the TA-DAs I find mine on Amazon.com (I am an Amazon junkie ☺) or you can find them on livinghands.net in our online store.

- 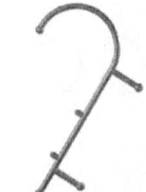 Theracane
- 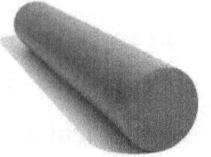 Foam Roller
- 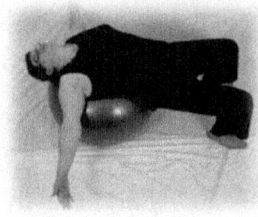 Exercise ball
- 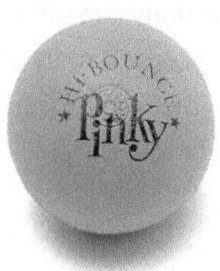 Pinky Ball (firmer than tennis ball)

CHAPTER 1
TYPES OF PAIN

Types of Pain Management

Pain has so many definitions but there are really only two types of pain, Acute and Chronic.

Acute pain is defined as 'pain that comes on quickly, can be severe, but lasts a relatively short period of time. Acute pain is usually the result of disease, injury or inflammation of the tissues. It can usually be diagnosed and treated.

Chronic pain is described as 'pain that persists or progresses over a long period of time and is resistant to most medical treatment.'

Living in constant pain can hinder your life style and relationships at home, work, with friends and with yourself. Chronic pain can limit the way or ability to do even the most simple of daily routines, such as brushing your hair, doing dishes, going up and down steps and more.

In 2006 I was in a car accident that left me not being able to sit or stand for more than 10 minutes without my back and neck going into spasms. This chronic pain ended my 21 year career as a dental assistant and forced me, as a single woman, to find a new career that satisfied my desire to help others, work with my hands and earn a living. My Christian faith and prayer life lead me to a career in Massage Therapy.

During my nearly 10 years of practice as a Massage Therapist, I have studied and learned much about pain and how it affects everyone differently. For example, one person's pain may feel minor to them but major to someone else. This is due to the pain receptors in our brains and how they read the pain from the Central Nervous System. I have had many wonder how, with the pain I endure daily, I am able to function or even stand up. This is due to a couple of reasons, one is "survival mode" and second, because my brain takes longer to acknowledge the pain coming from the signal of my Nervous System.

Whether you live with acute pain or chronic pain, it is a major deal to you.

Rest assured my friends, there may be some very easy and simple ways to ease your pain before it takes complete hold of you.

Learning to read and listen to your body is a good start.

CHAPTER 2
TYPES OF PAIN MANAGEMENT

I have mentioned in Chapter 1 that there are many ways to manage your pain. In this book I will be sharing some of the natural options that I have found to be helpful to me and to my clients.

The first is learning to read and listen to your body. Your body will actually "tell" you that there is an issue before it becomes apparent.

Did you know that the muscles around an area of concern will tighten first with or mostly without any pain? Then the achiness begins, but we just continue going and going until "WHAM!" the pain hits. Taking steps at the tight muscle stage can help ward off the final pain stage.

Here are some examples, if you wake up in the morning and are still tired but had plenty of time to sleep this could indicate that the deeper muscles close to the bone are inflamed and/or tightened onto the nervous system, usually in about four to five days you will feel the outer muscles very tight and/or pain. Another is if you feel a burning, tingling, or sharp pain while working out you have over stretched the muscle fibers which will most likely result in very sore muscles causing compensation or an injured muscle. It is good to feel the burn but there is also a limit that most of us ignore causing damage, and then we just "work" through it not realizing that scar tissue is forming. Once scar tissue is present there is only one way to remove it and that is surgery. However, there are ways to work with the muscle fibers to turn it into a flexible scar.

Scar tissue will hinder to function of the muscle. It will not allow the muscle to perform fully causing compensation to the surrounding muscles or muscles of the opposite side. Some of the outside natural treatments listed below can help with is condition.

     Over the years I have monitored my clients and have found that most of their chronic pain or recurring pain is due to the area of the body being over worked, poor posture, compensation for an old injury, or poor sleeping habit (such as stomach sleeping).

Before looking into any of these outside natural options **consult your physician first.**

Here are some of the methods I use and have shared with my clients.

MASSAGE THERAPY: is the

scientific manipulation of the soft tissues of the body for the purpose of normalizing those tissues and consists of manual techniques that include applying fixed or movable pressure, holding and/or causing movement of or to the body.

I will share in this book the techniques I practice but keep in mind there are numerous methods of massage therapy these are just a few.

These forms of Massage Therapy are effective on back pain (both upper and lower), carpal tunnel symptoms, sciatica, hip pain, headaches (including migrains), plantar fasciitis, tendonitis, knee pain and much more.

NEUROMUSCULAR THERAPY: is a manual precise protocol that applies pressure in a perpendicular manner to the skin surface to stimulate the muscle release.

TRIGGER POINT THERAPY: is a manual therapy whereas the Therapist applies direct pressure to the belly of the muscle and holds it for several seconds. However, I have found that surrounding the tightened muscle with several pressure points is more effective and more comfortable to the client.

CRANIOSCACRAL THERAPY: is an alternative therapy that uses a gentle touch to manipulate the cranium, spine or pelvic. This technique works with the flow of the cerebrospinal fluid to aid in the release of stress and tension.

LYMPHATIC DRAINAGE: is a gentle, rhythmic style of massage that mimics the action of the lymphatic system. This technique uses precise rhythm and pressure to open the initial lymphatic and to stimulate lymph vessels to contract. This helps with edema. However, not all therapists are trained in the advanced LDT so you will need a Certified LDT therapist that is trained to help with more advanced issues such as extreme edema and cancer.

ORTHOPEDIC MASSAGE: Is a form of massage that addresses orthopedic conditions from the perspective of treatment, prevention or rehabilitation. Orthopedic massage includes a wide range of soft tissue modalities to treat conditions resulting from a number of activities, like work, sports or accidents. This type of massage addresses the pain or injury affecting the locomotors soft tissue, such as the joints, skeleton, muscles, fascia, ligaments, tendons or cartilage. This is a great one for sprains, strains or pulled muscles.

DEEP TISSUE: Is the modality that uses specific techniques and pressure that releases the deeper tissue. This technique is slower and precise in its application. It can sometimes be uncomfortable but it is not always necessary. Deep Tissue Therapy just means you get into and release the deepest layer at the bone. Pain is not always needed to achieve this.

AROMATHERAPY: This is the use of essential therapeutic grade oils in a controlled environment. The use of essential oils are on the most part safe, but if uses improperly can lead to major health issue. **CAUTION: use only with the guidance of a medical professional or certified aromatherapist.**

HOT STONE: is a specialty massage where the therapist uses smooth, heated stones to help relax the nervous system and tight muscles.

CRYOTHERAPY: is the use of heat or cold to reduce inflammation and/or relax muscle tissues.

INFRARED THERAPY: also known as **PHOTOTHERAPY** is the use of LED controlled light for a specific period of time to warm the injured or inflamed tissue to help speed healing. This is a great treatment for relaxing tight muscles and easing pain.

COMPRESSIONS: the use of moist heat pack or cold packs on the affected areas of inflammation or injury.

TOPICAL APPLICATIONS: there are multiple OTC topical analgesics out there. Again, the product that works for you may not work on someone else. The two I have found to be most beneficial are Biofreeze and Sombra warming gel.

CHIROPRACTIC:

is a health care profession concerned with the diagnosis, treatment and prevention of disorders of the neuro-musculoskeletal system and the effects of these disorders on general health. It is a science, art and philosophy of locating and correcting problematic areas in the nervous system.

According to Dr. Shawn M. Pala, Chiropractic Physician (since 2006) of Pala Chiropractic located in Noblesville, Indiana; chiropractic treatment can help manage pain by:

- placing emphasis on the patient recuperative abilities rather than surgery,

- recognize that dynamics exist between lifestyle, environment and health

- understanding the cause of illness in order to eliminate it, rather than treating just the symptoms

- focusing on early intervention by placing emphasis on timely diagnosis and treatment of conditions that are wholly functional and reversible

- keeping the treatment patient-centered.

There are many different chiropractic techniques, such as:

- **High velocity low amplitude** adjustments which use quick but firm manipulations. This style provides immediate feeling of relief by the "joint popping" of the spine that some prefer.

- **Low-forced technique** is a style preferred by others.

- **Logan Basic** is one of the lowest-forced techniques which uses a light, sustained force exerted against a specific contact point on the sacrum and the base of the spine. The doctor uses light pressure (about 2 ounces) on auxiliary contact points along the spine and specific muscles from the base of the lower back to the head. Using the muscular structure surrounding the sacrum as a lever system, the entire structure of the spine can be balanced. Logan Basic is a safe treatment for muscular spasms, acute injuries and post-surgical pain. Logan Basic can be safely administered in the treatment of previous laminectomy (removal of the back of one or more vertebrae) or fusion of the cervical or lumbar spine.
Logan Basic uses no manipulation of the spine.

Tools used in chiropractic treatments can be helpful in achieving ultimate results. These include specific tables that are equipped with adjustable cushions allowing treatment to be more comfortable.

Dr. Pala states that the use of the Activator Method (an adjusting instrument), Kinesiotaping (taping of muscles to aid in providing support while the body works on the inflammation in a specific area) and Transcutaneous Electrical Stimulation (TENS) of the muscles are an important part of the patient treatment.

Relief with chiropractic treatment depends on the length of time the conditions has lasted and other factors such as age, health conditions(such as rheumatoid or osteoarthritis, lupus, diabetes or other degenerative conditions).

Chiropractic patients enjoy their treatments and look forward to returning.

Chiropractic treatments usually are between 15 – 30 minutes after the initial visit which can be up to 2 hours.

Most insurance policies cover chiropractic treatment. Checking with your insurance company prior to your visit would help you be prepared for any deductibles, co-pays or any limitations, or checking with your Chiropractor to see if they offer verifying of your benefits for you.

NUTRITION:

We all know that food plays a huge part of our health; however, did you know that it can play a major part of your pain?

Today our food is loaded with chemicals to preserve and modify it from its original state to increase productivity. These chemicals have been proven to destroy tissue and molecular structures of our bodies systems, thus causing disease and illness.

    Over the last few years I have learned much about what foods can help with my pain management, as well as the proper food combinations. Yes that is what I said, food combinations. According to Catherine Rudolph, Certified Nutritionist, Owner of Food That Heal You and Author, eating improper food combinations cause the foods that metabolize faster to become fermented in our digestive systems and can cause multiple issues due to the foods eaten at the same time that metabolize slower.

    In her book "Foods That Heal" Catherine addresses detailed information on healthy food choices (and unhealthy food choices) to help you obtain and maintain a healthy lifestyle.

Her book also includes a proper food combining chart, and over 50 quick healthy recipes using proper food combining principles to help heal digestion and maximize weight loss.

    I am learning that a happy gut is a healthier me.

CHAPTER 3

TA-DAs

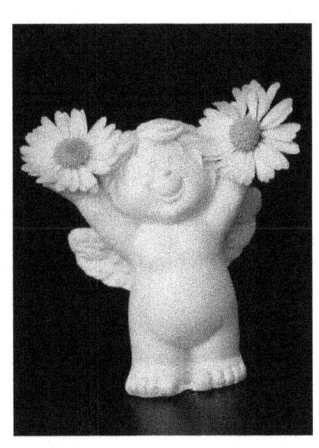

TA-DAs

Now comes the fun part, the sharing of my pain management TA-DAs. In this section, I will be sharing the techniques, supplements, essential oils and nutritional TA-DAs I use on myself or clients have shared that has helped manage daily chronic pain.

Keep in mind a technique is not for everyone but may just be the one that gives you the TA-DA you need to live a more comfortable and enjoyable life.

> **NOTE: I have found if my muscles are extremely tight pain medication or muscle relaxants only take the edge off and manual manipulation from a professional healthcare provider is what helps the most.**

LOWER BACK

Lower back or back pain period can be a pain in itself and can be caused by a number of reasons. The most common are improper posture, disc issues (such as herniated or bulging), and injury, overuse, degeneration of vertebrae, impingement of a nerve, or disease such as cancer, MS, spondylosis, etc.

Chronic back pain makes bending over to even put on your sock and shoes a chore, let alone standing in lines, sitting at your desk, standing to do the dishes, walking , going up and down steps, lifting or even playing with your children or grand babies.

When the pain from improper posture, overuse, broken coccyx (tailbone), degeneration of vertebrae and the turning of vertebra, whiplash scar tissue, fibromyalgia and the aftermath of mold poisoning hit me I was bound and determined to find natural pain relief and management. Like a lot of you, I prefer not to put chemical pain medications into my body that can, with long term use, be harmful to the liver and kidneys or become addictive if at all possible. The TA-DAs I will share are how I help keep myself going day by day when the medical community is wondering how.

QUADRATUS LUMBORUM, PIRIFORMIS & PSOAS

The **Quadratus Lumborum (QL)** is a deep muscle that can cause pain that radiates into the gluts and is located in the back at the waistline.

The QL tilts the pelvic and flexes the spine to the side.

Pain in the QL includes the lower back and into the gluts.

The **Piriformis** is a deep muscle of the gluteus.

The Piriformis helps to rotate the hips outward and bring it inward when flexed.

A tight Piriformis muscle can cause low back pain at the waistline area, in the gluts, down the leg, and into the toes due to the compression of the sciatic nerve.

The **Psoas** is the middle layer of the gluteus.

The Psoas major helps to flex the hip and rotate it outward and bringing it inward. The Psoas minor tilts the pelvic backward (sway back)

The Psoas can cause pain in the lower back, the front of the hips and thigh and into the belly button area.

I have discovered some fairly simple methods to release these muscles on my own. I call them the **QL release** and **Piriformis release** and the **Psoas release**. Pretty fancy names, don't you think?

QL RELEASE

- This is done while you are standing with feet hip distance apart placing your hands on your hips with your thumbs next to your spine (not on the spine, but next to it).
- Then squeeze in toward the spine and press down toward floor at the same time.
- Hold this position until you feel the back relax. You should feel your hips moving and your back unwinding.

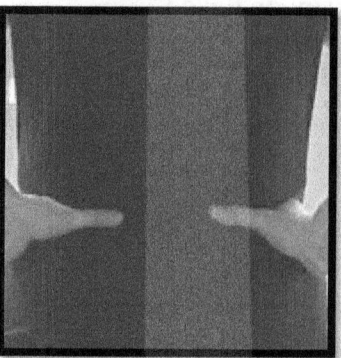

The use of a foam roller horizontally is also a great QL release.

- Lay on the foam roller at the lower back, face up.
- Slowly roll the roller up the back until you reach the shoulders or neck.
- Where it is tender or extra tight I usually just hang there for a few extra seconds.

- You may also feel or hear some "crunchies" this is ok.

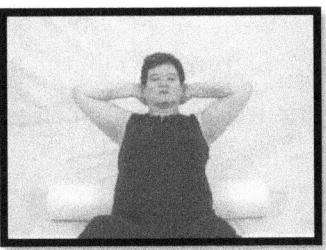

PIRIFORMIS RELEASE

This is best achieved laying down on the floor but can also be done on the bed or sitting on a hard chair.

- Laying on your back place a tennis ball, golf ball or I prefer a pinky ball (much firmer than a tennis ball) or a client suggested dogs chew ball the size of the tennis ball or your fist if none of the above are available, under you at the back pocket area. You will know you are there for it will be a little tender. If it is too tender move the ball a little up toward waist or a bit out toward the hip.
- Bend your knee (the side the ball is on) foot flat on the floor
- Very slowly move your knee inward. When you feel it tender or pressure on the ball hold it. Within 2-5 seconds the pressure will ease and you can continue moving

inward until you hit another tight area. Once you have gone inward as far as you can, slowly move outward repeating the same pattern of release. Repeat if needed.
- Repeat sequence for the opposite side. You always want to balance yourself out.

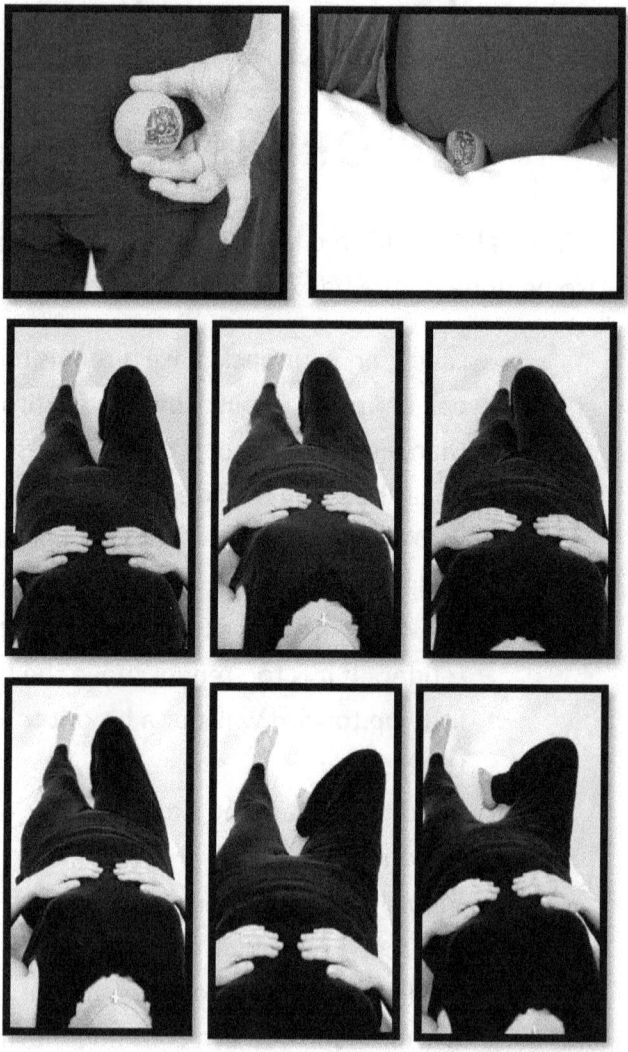

PSOAS RELEASE

This one works best done laying face up

- Laying face up cup your fingers over hipbone resting the palm of your hand on the outside of the hip. This can be done legs flat or knees bend.
- Gently pull fingers outward while pressing in with the palm of the hand.
- Hold until you feel the lower back relaxing.

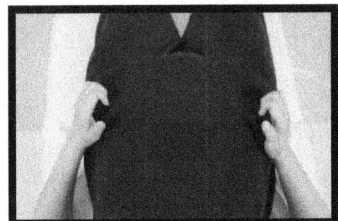 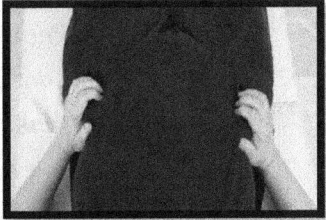

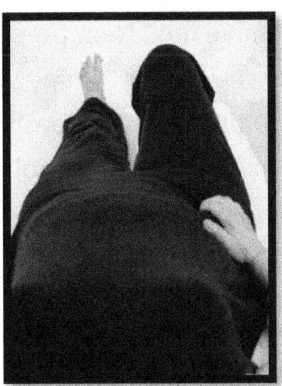

TA-DA at this point your lower back, toosh, and hips should feel relaxed and loving you.

SHOULDERS

Ah! Those beautiful shoulders, they take a lot of beating.

Shoulder issues can come in many different forms and reasons, such as injury, overworking, postural, disease, tightened muscles.

> **NOTE:** *Did you know that between your shoulder blades is the cutaneous referral point to your stomach? Yep, when the muscles of the upper shoulder tighten it may increase the issues with acid reflux, IBS, and other digestive issues.*

Don't believe me. Next time you are getting your massage see if your tummy starts making noise when the therapist is releasing your shoulders. It is a fun experiment and cool TA-DA. So, with this fun knowledge let's see how we may be able to help those awesome shoulders.

Let's start by looking at the rotator cuff muscles.

There are four rotator cuff muscles that can pose many issues. They are the Supraspinatus, Subscapularis, Infraspinatus, and Teres minor.

SUPRASPINATUS

The **supraspinatus** is located at the top of the shoulder.

The supraspinatus helps the arm move outward.

Tightening of this muscle can cause pain that radiates down the outside of the arm to the thumb with pain or tightness in the upper arm (the deltoids) you may have trouble raising your arm. So, here is a TA-DA that just might help.

I find closing my eyes and breathing slowly and evenly help my body to respond quicker.

- Grab hold of your collar bone (DO NOT press into it).
- Pull down toward your feet (NOT into the body).
- I hold until the top of the shoulders ease.

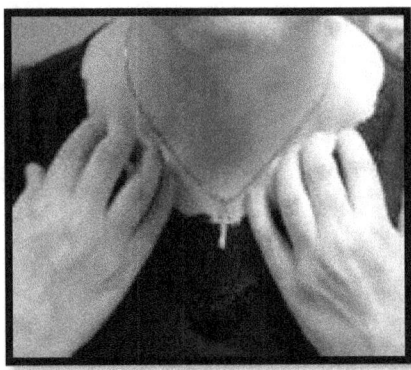

You should feel the top of your shoulder releasing. TA-DA!

INFRASPINATUS

The **infraspinatus** is a large triangular muscle that covers most of the shoulder blade.

It helps to rotate the arm and stabilize the shoulder joint.

When this muscle is overused or injured, pain is noticed in the upper arm, shoulder blade close to the spine and radiates down the arm on the inside and outside to the top /palm of the hand.

I have found the best TA-DA to release this on my own has a couple of ways.

- Place a tennis ball on your shoulder blade while up against a wall.
- Press into the ball.
- Bring opposite hand to shoulder and press against the wall.
- Sometimes I rock back and forth on it.

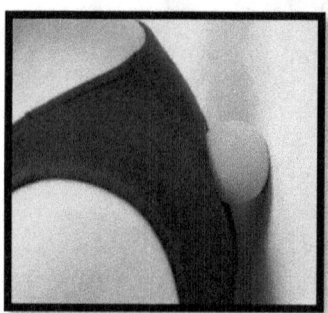 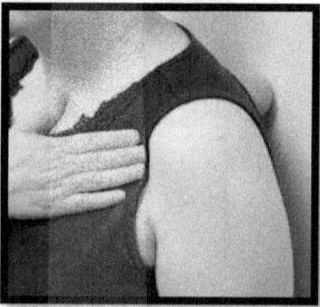

The second option:

- Lay face up on the floor.
- Place ball under the shoulder in the middle of the shoulder blade.
- Rest arm out to side.
- Bring opposite hand to shoulder and press into the floor.
- Hold – it usually releases in about 20-60 seconds.

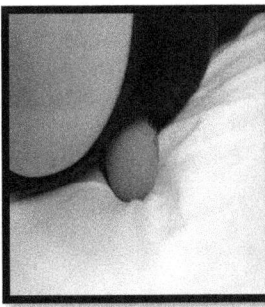 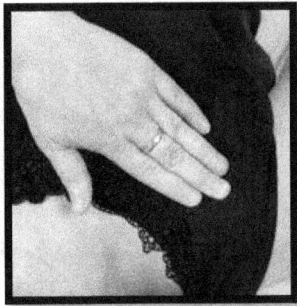

Third option:

- Lay face up on an exercise ball balancing or foam roller, at the upper back and shoulders.
- Stretch your arms out to the side and hold.

This stretches the pectoralis muscles and thus helps to release the infraspinatus.

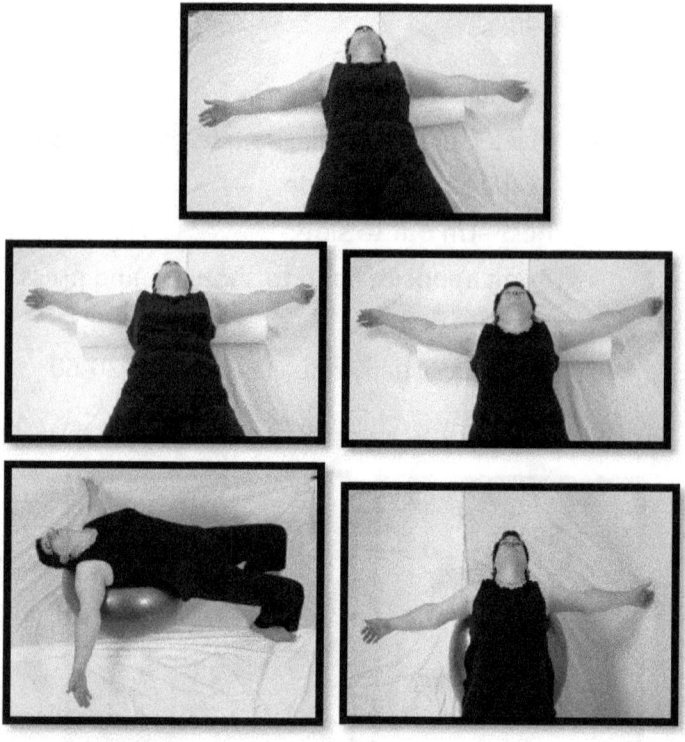

SUBSCAPULARIS

AH! The **Subscapularis** muscle. This is what I call the big trouble maker. It is the muscle under the shoulder blade. It will tighten up the whole shoulder, the upper arm (delts), the pec, the neck, the lats and it thinks because it is hidden it cannot get releases, but TA-DA.

This one is more difficult to do on your own but can be done. The use of a Theracane or any other pressure point cane can help with this one.

- Lay face up on floor (is best) or bed

- Bring your opposite arm across your body
- With the first three fingers slide down the breast line on the side **(DO NOT GO UP INTO THE ARMPIT)**
- Press inward and you should feel a ledge
- Pressing in and down toward the floor/bed hold until release

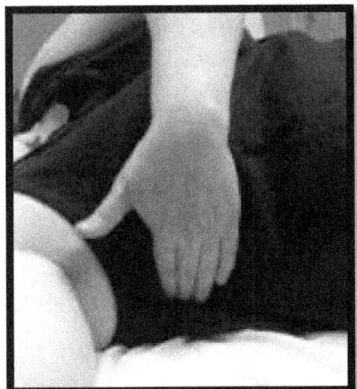
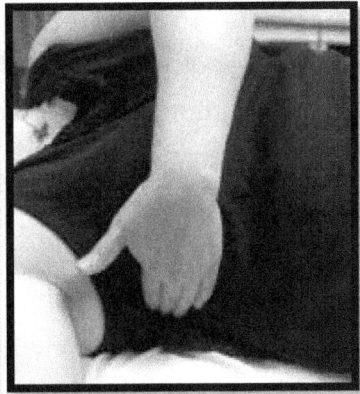
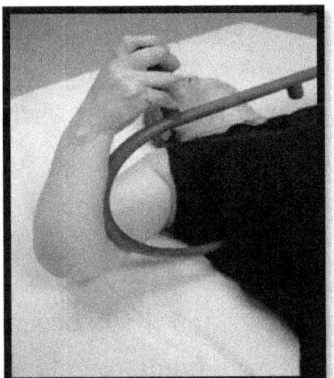

When the **subscapularis** is releasing I can feel my shoulder relax and my back unwinding (relaxing).

DIGESTIVE SYSTEM

I mentioned before that the digestive system can be inhibited by the tightness of the shoulders, however, this is not always the case.

There are many reasons for digestive issues such as IBS, Crohn's disease, and Ulcerated Colitis, a missing Gallbladder, improper nutrition, stress as well as others.

Here are some TA-DAs that have helped me and several of my clients regulate their digestive issues.

These TA-DAs involves a little valve that connects the small intestine to the large intestine. It is located on the right side slightly above the hip bone. This valve is called the **Ileocecal valve** and it can cause some uncomfortable situations. When the Ileocecal valve is stuck open, you have loose bowels. When it is stuck closed, you are constipated. Both issues may cause bloating, inflammation, irritability and if not dealt with diseases.

The **large intestine release** and **the Ileocecal Valve release** are some of the ways I have found to help with digestive issues.

The digestive system work **RIGHT TO LEFT ALWAYS!**

I tell my client to remember the Pledge of Allegiance- right hand to left chest.

ILEOCECAL VALVE

- Lay on floor or bed face up.
- **REMEMBER THE RIGHT** HIP BONE AREA place three to four fingers along the inside of hip bone slightly pointing upward toward belly button.
- With a light to moderate pressure (the feel of a quarter or apple) press down toward the floor, then slightly toward the belly button.
- When this releases, move slightly toward the belly button and repeat sequence. The release may be felt as muscle movement or as pressure releasing. I sometimes feel a little tender here.
- Continue until you have reached your belly button.

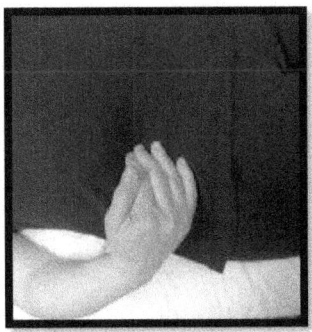 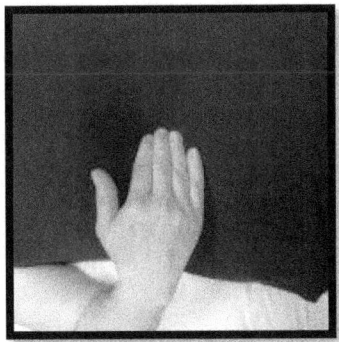

TA-DA! This should work fairly quickly. I usually have relief within 45 minutes, but sometimes have to repeat for a couple of days especially if mine has been closed for a while.

DIGESTIVE RELEASE

This TA-DA has a couple of ways to release.

First option:

- Sitting down is best.
- **ALWAYS RIGHT TO LEFT** and hip bone, belly button, hip bone. Grab with both hands the tummy by the RIGHT hip bone.
- Lift up.
- Slightly pull LEFT hand toward belly button
- You should feel a release or relaxation of the muscles quickly.
- Move RIGHT hand to meet the LEFT and move LEFT hand about one inch toward belly button.
- Continue this sequence until you have reached the LEFT hip bone.

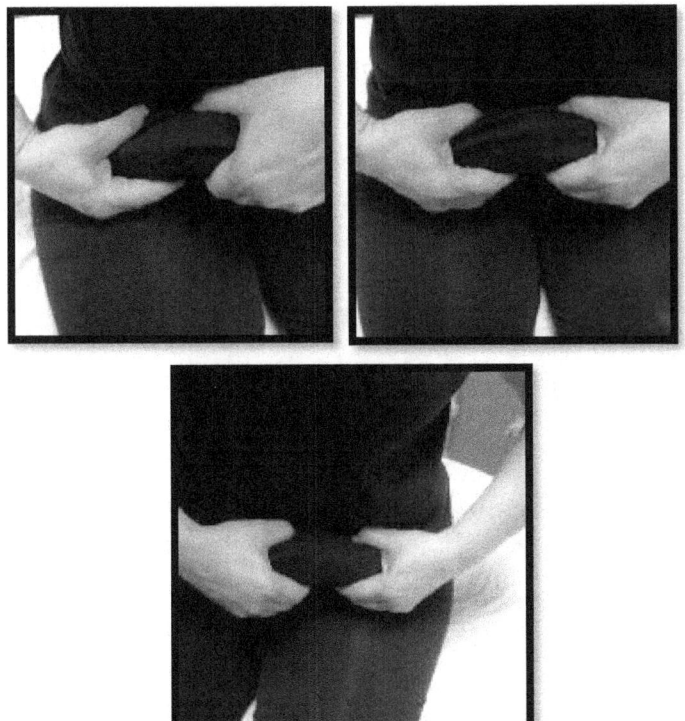

You may feel a "Knot" at times, this is the foods that are not digesting quickly or properly so this helps move it along. I have found on many occasions that within 45 minutes I am cleansing out. Enough said there☺.

If you feel tightness at the "V" of the ribs and having digestive issues this may be a twist in the large intestines. **However, make sure you do not have a hernia in this area.**

- Lay on your back.
- Find your belly button and two fingers up.

Pain Management TA-DAs

- Press down toward the floor/bed until you feel your heart beat and slightly up toward your ribs.
- I usually hold for about 30 seconds. You should feel a release or relaxation of the muscles.
- **SLOWLY** with your breath release the hold of the fingers and TA-DA.

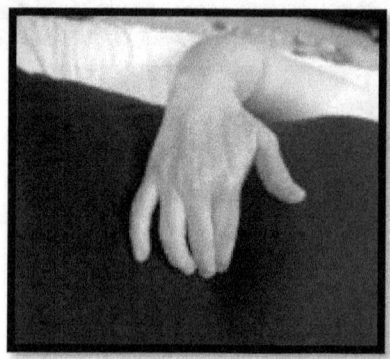

One of my colleagues taught me this one. ☺

BREATHING

JUST BREATHE
JUST BREATHE
JUST BREATHE
JUST BREATHE

Many of us do not realize that under our everyday stresses whether good ones or bad ones, our back and rib muscles tighten. This tightness decreases our breathing range, meaning we begin to breathe shallower without even knowing it. Breathing shallowly reduces the oxygen we intake, thus decreasing the oxygen to the major organs and the brain. Here are some TA-DAs to help you 'Just Breathe".

NOTE: With these releases if you do not feel the relaxations lighten up on the pressure. When releasing intercostals, (rib) muscles the less pressure the better.

RIB RELEASE

- Sitting upright place your first finger between the ribs just under the breast and allow the thumb to rest between the ribs in the back.
- Gently press in toward the front then slightly downward.
- Hold until you feel a relaxation.
- Breathing slowly and deep.
- Keeping hands in the same position now press backward and slightly down.
- Hold until you feel a relaxation.
- Breathing slowly and deep.

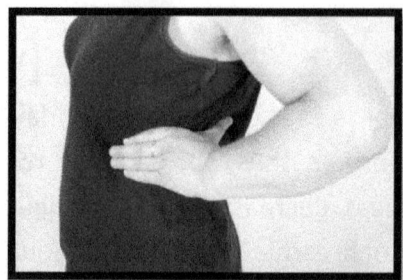
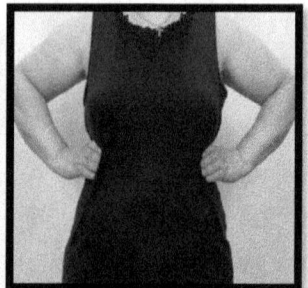
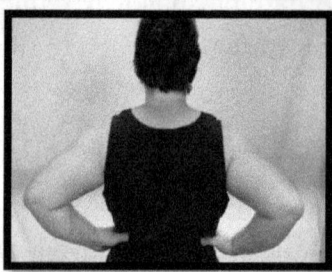

At this point, you should be able to notice an easier breathing as well as a little release in the mid back.

Using the same sequence let's relax the chest area. This TA-DA is really great when you are congested.

- Sitting upright place your first three (3) fingers on both sides of the sternum (breast bone) between the ribs.
- Gently press inward toward the middle and slightly downward.
- Hold until you feel a relaxation.
- Breathing slowly and deep.

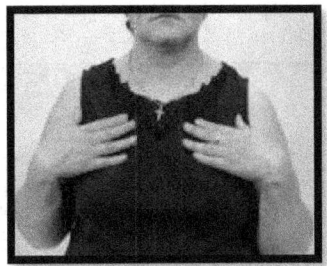

Here if you feel a tightness or "knot", it could be congestion plug. **However, if it does not release seek medical evaluation to rule out any serious issues.**

CHEST/THROAT RELEASE

This TA-DA is very helpful when you have a nagging, tickling cough.

- Cupping your first three (3) fingers and the thumb together place them in the middle of the chest.
- Press inward then gently twist clockwise.
- Reverse and twist counter clockwise.
- The same sequence can be done at the "Adam's Apple" area for a tickle in the throat.

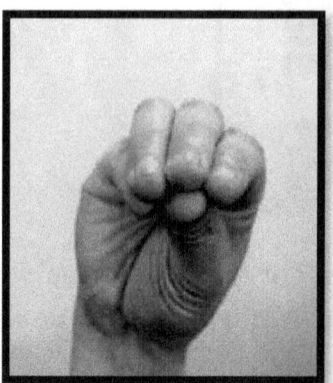 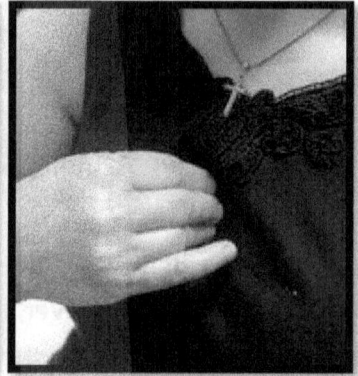

TA-DA this should relax the muscles that are in a spasm

TMJ/TMD

The Temporomandibular Joint is the joint that joins the lower jaw to the upper. It is located just in front of the ears. This joint is tough but when it is inflamed or damaged it can cause much pain.

The pain path for the Temporomandibular Joint affects the back of the head, around the eyes, the forehead above the eyebrow, the joint area in front of the ears, and down the neck.

> **Did you know that there is a direct connection to teeth clenching or grinding and your hip placement? We all have the tendency to lean or favor one side. The jaw being on a hinge slides to the same side causing the teeth not to mesh properly and putting pressure on the TMJ joint. The teeth don't like to be out of alignment, so we find ourselves clinching and grinding to get back into alignment.**

The TA-DAs I will show you to release your jaw are not pretty and can feel odd but it really works.

EXTERNAL TMJ RELEASE

First one is releasing the outside of the jaw.

- Bringing the fingers of the opposite hand to the "V" of the jaw, just in front of the earlobes, and the fingers of the other hand just below the top fingers on the jaw bone.
- Gently press inward and slightly down on the lower fingers and up with the upper fingers, allowing your jaw to relax open slightly.
- Hold until it relaxes.
- Continue with this sequence following the jaw line.

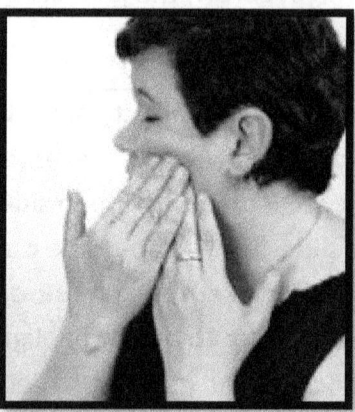

Second option:
- Place the fingers of the hand of same side on the "V" of the jaw.
- Bring the opposite fingers just underneath the top hand at the lower jaw.
- Gently press inward, separating the hands slightly.
- Hold until it releases.

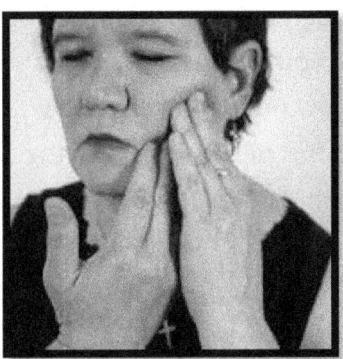

INTERNAL TMJ RELEASE

The second one is a little messier but will release both the outside and inside at the same time.

- Using the middle finger of the opposite hand and the first three fingers of the other hand, open mouth enough to get the middle finger in alongside the cheek (you will feel a muscle at the back where the upper jaw meets the lower jaw).
- Placing the first three fingers of the other hand at the outer junction of the jaw (just in front of the earlobe).
- Together, at the same time, press the inside finger and the outer fingers together and slightly downward.
- Hold until it relaxes.
- Follow the jaw line all the way out to the lips (swallowing as needed but keeping fingers in place) keeping the jaw relaxed and slightly open.
- Repeat for the opposite side.

TA-DAs

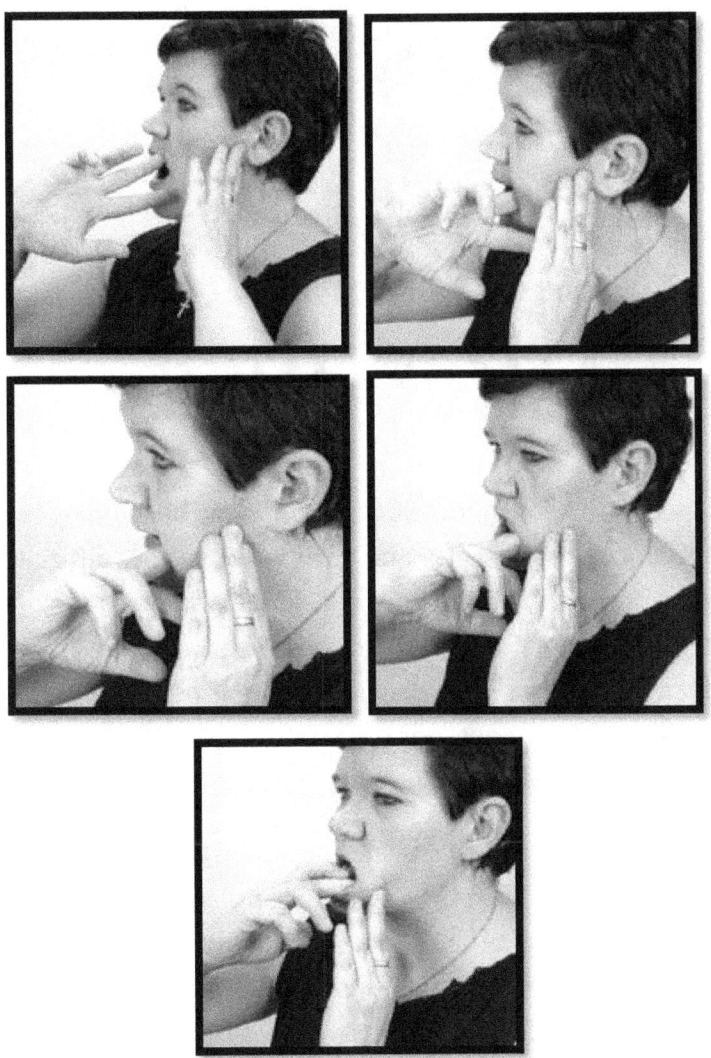

TA-DA you should have a relaxed jaw, eased temples and easier opening of the mouth.

HEADACHES & MIGRAINES

I don't know about you but when my head hurts everything seems off kilter and it can become very difficult to function. **If you suffer from repeated headaches seek medical attention immediately.** After seeking medical assistance and have been diagnosed with tension, sinus headaches or migraines, here are some TA-DAs that might lessen the duration or prevent the onset.

Some headaches may be caused by the tightening of a neck muscle called the **Levator Scapulae** which attached to the top of the shoulder to the base of the head. When this muscle tightens, it can enhance the pressure behind the eyes and at the base of the head. This can cause sinus pressure headaches or migraine style headaches. It can also come across with pain in and around the shoulder blade or top of the shoulder.

Clenching and Grinding of the teeth can also result in headaches at the base of the head and in the temple area.

Go to the TMJ/TMD TA-DAs to help with your headaches or you can try these TA-DAs.

NECK RELEASE

- Placing your fingers on the back of your neck in the groove next to the spine (pinky finger will be up against the base of the head).
- Press fingers inward toward the spine.
- Going clockwise (in toward spine and upward then outward) in a circular motion (I found rotating slowly provides more relief).
- Pause, keeping fingers in position reverse the circular motion and go counter clockwise (in toward spine then down and out).
- Continue moving your fingers down the neck, repeating the sequence until the index finger is resting on the top of the shoulders.
- Moving back up to the base of the head, slightly move fingers away from the spine about 2 fingers width.
- Repeat sequence.
- Continue moving fingers and repeating sequence until you come to just under the ears.

Pain Management TA-DAs

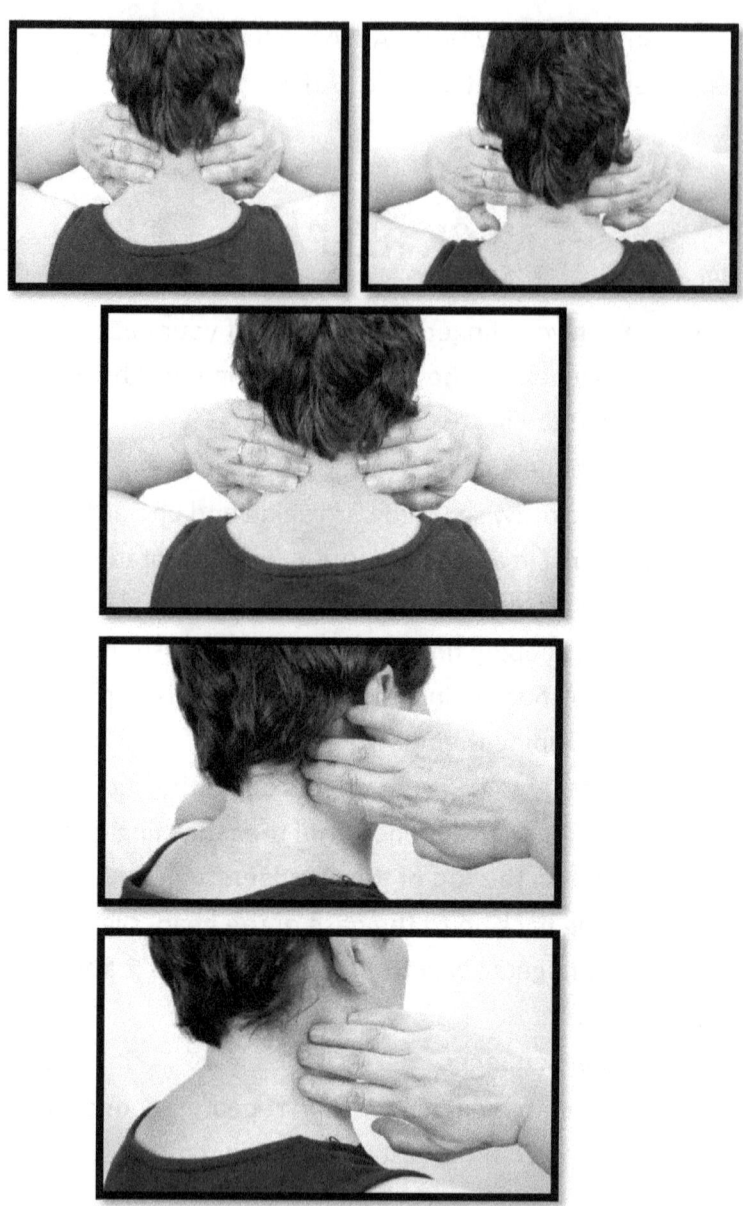

50

TA-DAs

There are some **pressure points** that help with headaches also:

#1

- Between the thumb and first finger in the webbing.
- Squeeze together and pull out at the same time.
- Hold until it relaxes.

#2

- Between the big toe and second toe on the top between the bones about 1" from the webbing.
- Press or use circular motion to stimulate.

#3

- Two fingers width from base of head there is a hollow between the muscles.
- Press or use circular motion to stimulate.

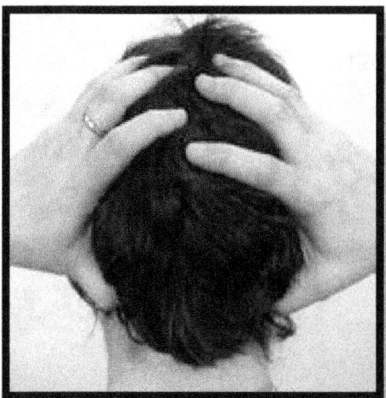

#4 sinus headaches

- Just above the eye brow.
- Temple areas (just outside the eye).
- Between the eye at the bridge of the nose.
- The outer sides of the nostrils near the bottom of the cheekbone.
- Press or circular motions to release.

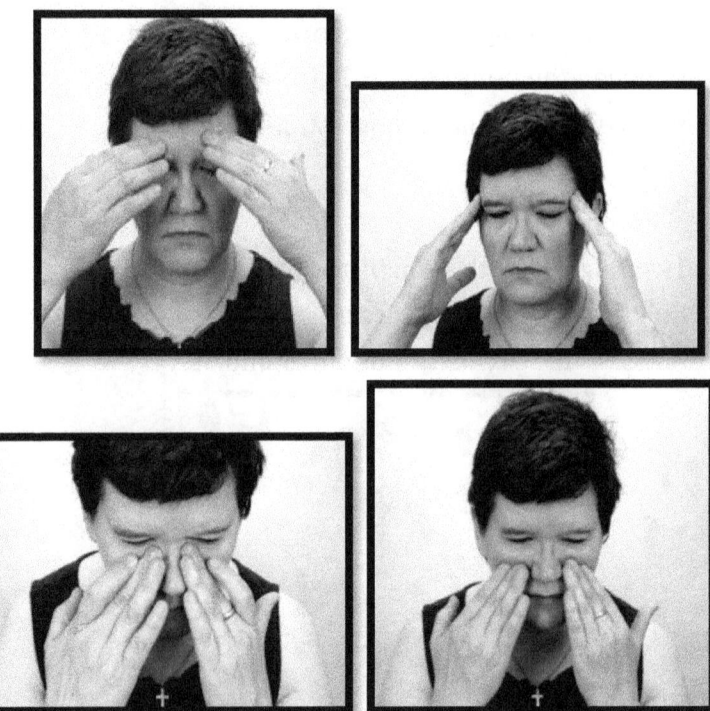

FEET

Oh, our poor feet! They take such a beating in just normal everyday life and when they complain life is not pleasant.

One of the major issues with the feet is **plantar fasciitis**. The plantar fascia is a membrane that covers the soles of the feet. Plantar fasciitis is usually associated with the tightening of the outer lower leg called the **peroneus longus** that attaches to the outer knee, wraps around the front of the ankle and inserts into the middle of the sole of the foot. When this muscle tightens, it takes with it the fascia of the foot. This causes much pain on the top of the foot and around the ankle. You can have difficulties while walking or stepping.

These TA-DAs have helped me stay stepping many of times.

PLANTAR FASCIA RELEASE: BOTTOM OF THE FOOT

NOTE: RELEASING THE PLANTAR FASCIA IS NOT COMFORTABLE BUT VERY EFFECTIVE.

- Sitting down, bring your foot over your opposite knee. Or if you are really flexible, sit on the floor and bend forward to grab hold of the foot.
- Bring the thumbs of both hands to the middle of the sole of the foot, or the fingers if you are bending forward.
- Pull thumbs/fingers away from each other toward the outside of the foot using as much pressure as you can tolerate.
- Hold pressure until it relaxes.
- Repeat the movement while moving the thumbs/fingers down toward the heel.

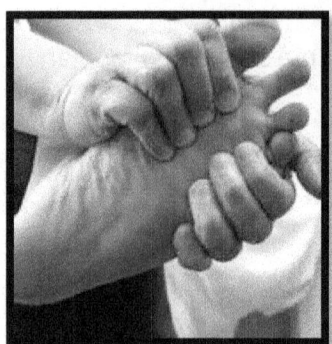 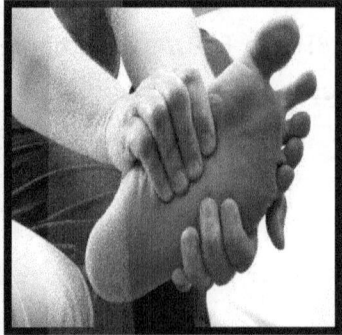

OR

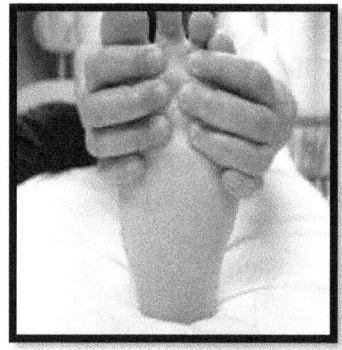 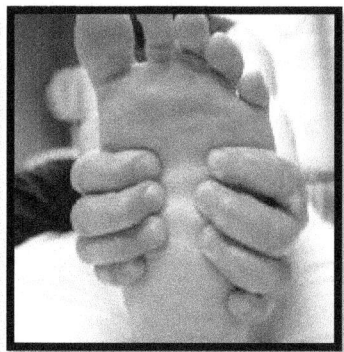

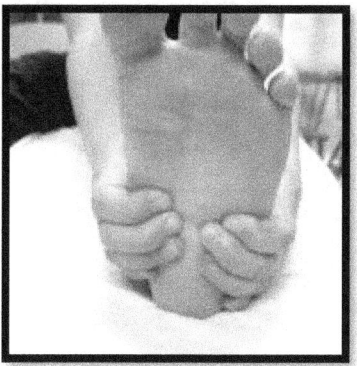

SECOND OPTION:

- Using a tennis ball, golf ball, pinky ball (a little harder than a tennis ball) or foot roller, roll the ball up and down on the foot.

For added release:

- Holding onto something sturdy such as a door knob, table, chair, place the ball on the bottom of the foot (I like to start at the ball of the foot).

- Lean onto the ball putting as much pressure as you can tolerate and slowly roll the ball up and down the sole of the foot.

HEEL PULL:

This TA-DA helps to relax the Achilles tendon.
- Crossing your ankle over your thigh.
- Grab hold of the back of your heal.
- Opposite hand holding onto the top of the ankle.
- Gently pull heel down and upper hand toward your knee.

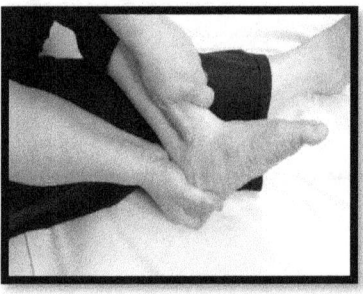

AGAIN THIS IS NOT COMFORTABLE BUT VERY EFFECTIVE!

Did you know that when the lower leg muscles tighten it may indicate a tight lower back that is causing the hip to rotate outward changing the way you walk on your feet?

HAND AND WRIST

Our hands and wrists are one of the most overworked parts of our bodies. With all the technology added to our everyday routines, injury and pain in these areas can become debilitating.

The pain in the hand, wrist, forearm and upper arm can limit our everyday duties, such as gripping a milk jug, cooking, grabbing up laundry, driving, computer work, brushing your hair, and more.

Let's look at one the most popular injuries, **Carpal Tunnel Syndrome.** In this syndrome, the carpal tunnel in the wrist becomes calcified blocking the flow of blood and pressing on the multiple nerves to the hand and fingers. Compensating for the pain, the forearm begins to tighten and then up the arm to the upper shoulder.

There are many other reasons for the hand, wrist, forearm and upper arm to be painful, tingling, or numb. For example, disc issues in the neck, over tight shoulder muscles or tennis elbow to name a few. There are also 8 carpal bones in the back of the wrist which can subluxate (partially dislocate). This condition can be treated by a chiropractor.

The causes are mainly overuse called **Repetitive Stress Syndrome,** where the muscle(s) are worked in the same position over and over until it becomes inflamed and painful. This syndrome can happen just about anywhere in the body, but mostly in the hand, wrist, lower back, shoulders, and neck.

I strongly urge you to seek medical advice if you have these symptoms to rule out "true" carpal tunnel. Advanced carpal tunnel syndrome is usually treated by surgery, although splinting, cortisone injections or essential oils may help ease the pain and inflammation.

As someone who uses her hands everyday in the workplace and with her hobbies of crocheting and gardening, I know this kind of pain.

Here are some of the TA-DAs I use for myself to continue in my busy pain management massage practice.

CARPAL TUNNEL RELEASE:

This TA-DA can be somewhat painful, but effective, so go slow and only to your comfort.

- With your opposite hand wrap your fingers around your wrist having the thumb on the underneath side.
- There will be three indentations. One on the thumb side, one In the middle of the wrist, and one on the outer side. I usually start on the thumb side.

- With the thumb of the opposite hand, using moderate pressure, press into the indentation.
- Hold for a few seconds then slowly inchworm up the groove to one inch below elbow **(DO NOT GO INTO THE CREASE OF THE ELBOW).**
- Repeat sequence in the middle and outer grooves.
- Turning your forearm over, repeat the sequence, to have the fingers underneath and the thumb on top.

> **The rice like knots are the fibers of the muscle all tangled up and can be the reason for the pain and inflammation. When I come to these, I hold my thumb there and rock back and forth a few times. I can feel them release and the pressure/pain ease.**

Pain Management TA-DAs

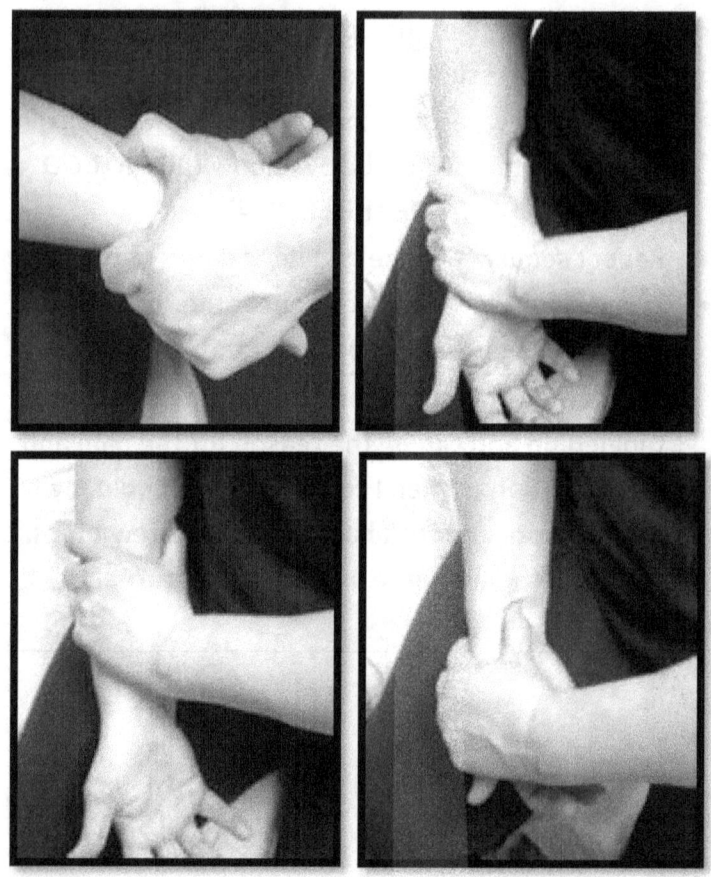

TA-DAs

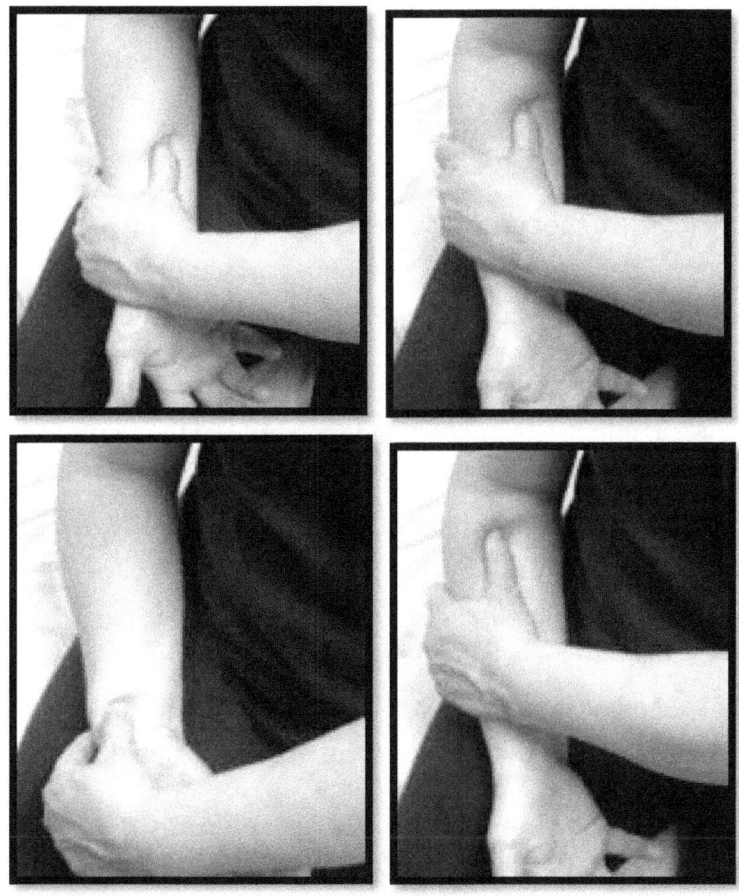

UPPER ARM RELEASE:

DELTOID RELEASE

The upper arm, also known as the **Deltoids,** are tight the pain covers the whole upper arm and can radiate down to the elbow on the outside. Here is the Deltoid Release TA-DA:

- Using the opposite hand grab hold of the upper arm /deltoid.
- Squeeze firmly but not too hard, and pull down toward the elbow.
- Hold until muscle relaxes (if it is not relaxing, lighten up on the pressure).
- Follow down the upper arm repeating the sequence to the end of the Deltoid / middle of upper arm.

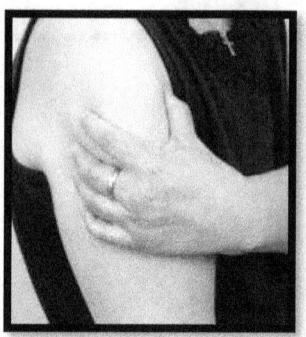
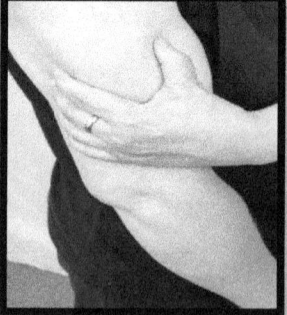

CHAPTER 4

ESSENTIAL OILS

ESSENTIAL OILS

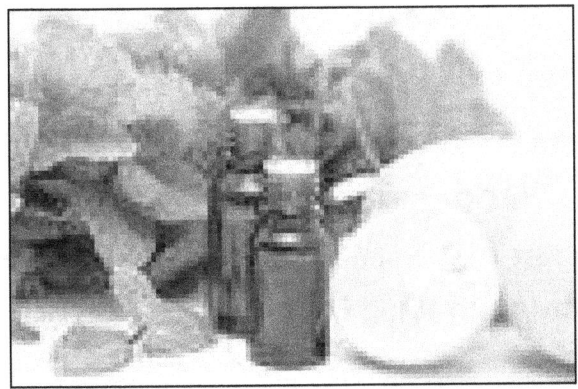

Essential Oils

I have found many essential oils to help in my pain management.

WARNING: DO NOT USE ESSENTIAL OILS WITHOUT THE GUIDANCE OF A HEALTHCARE PROFESSIONAL OR CERTIFIED AROMATHERAPIST

Aromatherapy has been around for centuries. Use of the entire plant, root, leaves, or flower in distilled processes can provide medicinal effects of the oil. This is why it is very important to use only with proper guidance. Essential oils can have as much effects on the body as prescription medication but with much less harm to major organs and less side effects.

There are many essential oils out there but to have the best results **undiluted therapeutic grade** oil is best. I have found the best ones are Eden's Garden, Young Living, and Doterra.

INFORMATION USED HERE ARE FROM THE "ESSENTIAL OILS OVERVIEW" by Mellissa M. Dawahare, ND, PLLC and the Center of Massage Therapy Continuing Education

And also the REFERENCE GUIDE FOR ESSENTIAL OILS APP.

Here are some that I use for pain management:

- **BLACK PEPPER**

Analgesic, anti-inflammatory, antiseptic, antispasmodic, antifungal, stimulates metabolism

HELP: obesity, fungal infections, sprains, rheumatoid arthritis, digestive and nervous system, arthritis, fatigue, muscle pain, increases adrenaline

CAUTION: avoid while pregnant, may cause extreme skin irritation

USE: topical: 1:1 dilution 2-4 drops on location.

Inhalation: in a diffuser very sparingly

- **FRANKINCENSE**

Antirumeral, antidepressant, immune booster, muscle relaxer, colds/coughs, digestion, inflammation, jaundice, respiratory issues, skin conditions.

HELP: cancer symptoms, respiratory infections, depression, inflammation, relaxation, stimulate pineal/pituitary glands/hypothalamus

CAUTION: Strong in scent, skin irritation

USE: topical: 1:1 dilutions apply 2-4 drops on location.

• HELICHRYSUM

Anesthetic, antispasmodic, liver protectant, liver detoxifier, liver stimulant, regenerates nerves

HELP: bruises, bone bruises, sciatica, tennis elbow, tinnitus, tissue repair, skin problems (dermatitis/eczema), burns, cholesterol, colitis, herpes simplex, arteriosclerosis, atherosclerosis

CAUTION: none

USE: topical: 1:1 dilutions apply 2-4 drops on location, temples, forehead, neck, or outer ear

Inhalation: directly or in diffuser for 15 minutes 2X daily

• LAVENDER

Antifungal, antiseptic, analgesic, anticonvulsant, antitumoral, vasodilator, anti-inflammatory, relaxant, cholesterol-lowering

HELP: nervous tension, insomnia, burns, scarring, stretch marks, eczema, psoriasis, insect bites, dermatitis, stress, respiratory infections,

infections, hypertension, PMS, menstrual problems, calming

CAUTION: none

USE: topical: direct apply 2-4 drops on location

Inhalation: directly or in diffuser for 15 minutes 2X daily

- ## **LEMONGRASS**

Anti-inflammatory, promotes lymph flow, improves circulation, regenerates ligaments and connective tissue

HELP: respiratory infections, sinus infections, bladder infections, digestive problems, salmonella, varicose veins, fluid retention, torn ligaments or muscles, carpal tunnel, whiplash, hyperthyroidism, cholesterol

CAUTION: breathing issues in persons with asthma, may cause extreme skin irritation

USE: topical: 1:4 dilutions (1 part oil to 4 parts carrier oil) apply 1-2 drops to location

Inhalation: direct or in a diffuser for 15 minutes 2X daily

• MYRRH

Antioxidant, antitumoral, antiparasitic, antiviral, analgesic, anesthetic, anti-inflammatory

HELP: Candida, ringworm, diabetes, cancer, hepatitis, eczema, tooth infections, gum infections, chapped/cracked skin, wrinkles, stimulates hypothalamus and pineal/pituitary glands.

CAUTION: Avoid while pregnant

USE: Topical: undiluted apply 2-4 drops on location.
Inhalation: direct/diffusion 15 minutes.

• MYRTLE

Liver stimulant, prostate and thyroid stimulant, antispasmodic, decongestant, anti-inflammatory

HELP: colds, bronchitis, thyroid problems, throat infections, sinus infections, lung infections, skin issues (acne, blemishes, bruises, psoriasis, oily skin), muscle spasms, prostate problems

CAUTION: none

USE: topical: 1:1 dilutions apply 2-4 drops on location

Inhalation: directly or in diffuser for 15 minutes 2X daily

- **ORAGANO**

Antibacterial, anti-inflammatory, immune stimulant, antispasmodic, antiseptic (to the respiratory system)

HELP: digestive problems, respiratory infections, arthritis, rheumatic disease

CAUTION: may irritate membranes of nasal passages, may cause extreme skin irritation.

USE: topical: 1:4 dilutions apply 1-2 drops on location

Inhalation: diffusion 15 minutes 2X daily

- **PEPPERMINT**

Anti-inflammatory, antibacterial, antifungal, antiparasitic, antiviral, analgesic, digestive stimulant, gallbladder stimulant

HELP: pneumonia, arthritis, digestive problems, headaches, nausea, dermatitis, eczema, psoriasis, scoliosis, back pain, lumbago

CAUTION: avoid while pregnant, do not use on children under 18 months old, and avoid contact with mucus membrane, sensitive skin, eyes, fresh wounds or burns

USE: topical: 1:1 dilution apply 1-2 drop on location, temples, abdomen

Inhalation: directly or in diffuser 15 minutes 2X daily

- **ROMAN CAMOMILE**

Antispasmodic, anti-inflammatory, relaxant, anesthetic, nerve regenerative, detoxifies blood and liver

HELP: restlessness, anxiety, ADHD< colitis, gastritis, insomnia, depression, skin problems (acne, eczema, dermatitis), PMS, stress, irritability, nervousness, muscle spasms, neuralgia

CAUTION: Avoid in pregnancy, can irritate sensitive skin

USE; topical: undiluted apply 1-2 drops on location, ankles, and wrists

Inhalation: direct or in diffuser for 15 minutes 2X daily

- **SPEARMINT**

Anti-inflammatory, antiseptic, increases metabolism, digestive aid, and gallbladder stimulant, antispasmodic

HELP: digestive problems, intestinal problems, obesity, headaches, bronchitis

CAUTION: avoid in pregnancy, not to be used on infants

USE: topical: 1:1 dilution apply 2-4 drops on location

Inhalation: directly or in diffuser for 15 minutes 2X daily

• TEA TREE

Antibacterial, anti-inflammatory, antifungal, antiparasitic, antiviral, antiseptic, decongestant, immune stimulant, tissue regeneration

HELP: Candida, sinus infection, lung infections, acne, skin sores, fluid retention, gum disease, hives, shingles, staph/MRSA, viral infections, wounds

CAUTION: repeated use may cause contact sensitization

USE: topical: 1:1 dilution apply 2-4 drops on location

Inhalation: directly or in diffuser for 15 minutes 2X daily

- **WINTERGREEN**

Anti-inflammatory, antispasmodic, anticoagulant, vasodilator, analgesic, anesthetic, antihypersensive

HELP: arteriosclerosis, fatty liver, arthritis, rheumatic disease, muscle pain, nerve pain, bone pain

CAUTION: avoid if epileptic, anticoagulant properties increase when used with warfain or aspirin

USE: topical: 1:1 (1 drop wintergreen to 1 drop carrier oil) apply 1-2 drops on location

Inhalation: directly or in diffuser for 15 minutes 2X daily

CHAPTER 5

HEALING FOODS AND HERBS

Pain Management TA-DAs

HEALING FOODS AND HERBS

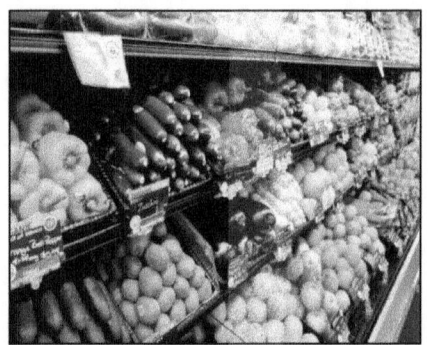

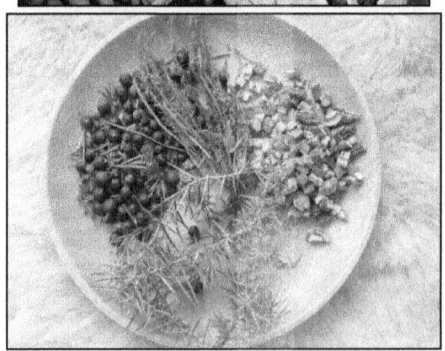

Many of us have missed out on the old time natural help that comes for the earth itself. Our food and plants have been contaminated with multiple chemicals that do not work with the delicate yet sturdy design of our bodies' natural rhythm thus causing illnesses and weaknesses.

Our bodies were created to heal itself, however with long term abuse illness and injuries happen and traditional medical treatment is necessary, but the addition of natural options to heal along with traditional options can allow us quicker healing and a more comfortable life.

I have found like many others that eating more organic, naturally raised foods have literally reduced my inflammation and pain levels, as well as eliminating or cutting down on gluten and refined sugars. This way of lifestyle has also helped in my digestive system which has been compromised by a missing gallbladder (which doctors do not tell you about) and the still detoxifying of the black mold poisoning from my system which can only be eliminated through the liver, kidney and urinary tract.

Here are some of the changes I have found helped me.

HEALING FOODS/HERBS

Listed are some of the foods I have increased in my eating lifestyle. They have the nutrients and vitamins that help to combat pain and inflammation.

FOR PAIN RELIEF:

- Coffee (limited to one cup daily)
- Salmon
- Ginger
- Turmeric
- Red grapes
- Thyme
- Cherries
- Cranberry juice (organic no sugar added)
- Herring
- Sardines
- Greek yogurt
- Mint tea
- Edamame
- Hot peppers
- Raspberries
- Red onions

- Tofu
- Kale
- Tuna
- Cabbage
- Green tea

FOR INFLAMMATION:

- Leafy greens (spinach, chard, kale)
- Fish (like wild caught salmon)
- Nuts
- Tomatoes
- Garlic and onions
- Berries
- Whole grains
- Olive oil
- Low fat dairy
- Beets
- Avocado
- Broccoli
- Carrots
- Dry beans
- Kale
- Bananas
- Oranges

- Sweet potatoes

HERBS FOR PAIN:

- Turmeric
- Ginger
- Valerian root
- Devil's claw
- White willow
- Licorice
- Oregano
- Fennel
- Clove
- Burdock
- Encomia

HERBS FOR INFLAMMATION:

- Turmeric
- Green tea
- White willow bark
- Martime pine bark
- Chili peppers
- Frankincense
- Black pepper
- Resveratrol

Pain Management TA-DAs

- Cat's claw
- Rosemary
- Cloves
- Cinnamon

CHAPTER 6

HERBAL SUPPLEMENTS

> **WARNING: DO TO THE MEDICIMAL PROPERTIES OF SOME HERBAL SUPPLEMENTS IT IS ADVISED TO CONSULT WITH YOUR MEDICAL PROFESSIONAL BEFORE TAKING ANY SUPPLEMENTS.**

HERBAL SUPPLEMENTS

We all get advice about supplements from our well intentioned friends and families, but really not all supplements are helpful. If used improperly they can become dangerous or not work at all if used inadequately.

According to Dr. Shawn M. Pala, Chiropractic Physician and owner of Pala Chiropractic in Noblesville, Indiana, the best supplements companies only allow licensed physicians to carry their products. These companies do extensive testing on their raw materials prior to manufacturing. Factors such as tablet disintegration time, mineral chelation, and absorption are studied. Whit minimal regulation of the supplement industry, purchases online can be fraudulent or harmful.

To determine what supplements are best for you Dr. Pala's office uses a symptom survey that will provide clinical information on cardiovascular, liver/biliary, thyroid, digestive, foundational and hormone imbalances. He also suggests blood work to help determine Vitamin D levels, liver enzymes, and complete blood counts to get the overall picture.

Patients can also use their Health Saving Accounts for supplements prescribed by their chiropractic physician when purchased in the doctor's office.

Julie Spencer resides in the Indianapolis, IN. area and was a dental assistant for 21 years before a car accident forced her to change careers.

Julie, with her strong Christian faith, was lead to the field of Massage Therapy, where she found a Gift that has helped her and many others suffering from chronic pain, for over ten years.

Julie lives with chronic pain daily due to old whiplash injuries, a broken tailbone, degenerative discs, osteoporosis, fibromyalgia, the aftermath of advanced mold poisoning, and scoliosis. Due to survival and her desire to manage her pain naturally; she was brought to writing this book of the TA-DAs that she does to herself. These allow her to be able to still garden, crochet, sit through concerts/plays (although not always easy), own and run her pain management massage practice and live life again.

Although Julie understands that her TA-DAs are not for everyone, she prays that you would be able to gain some relief and learn some natural options to managing your pain, plus gain some pep back into your step.

Find out more about Julie E Spencer, CMT, Author at: LH Pain Management Massage, LLC

lhpainmgmt.com   317-213-4523

REFERENCES

Julie E Spencer
LH Pain Management Massage, LLC
160 W. Carmel Drive
Suite 224
Carmel, IN. 46032
317-213-4523
lhpainmgmt.com
lhpainmanagementmassage@gmail.com

Dr. Shawn M. Pala, Chiropractic Physician
Pala Chiropractic
14701 Cumberland Road
Suite 350
Noblesville, Indiana 46060
317-770-1970
drshawnpala@gmail.com
www.palachiropractic.com
(Supplements, symptom testing & inserts for pelvic stabilizing)

Catherine Rudolph, CNC, Owner, Author
Foods That Heal You
Nationwide – based in Indianapolis, IN.
317-698-6150
Foodsthathealyou.com
Foodsthathealyou@gmail.com

Bill Spencer
INDY SKY PHOTOS
Photography for all your Special Events
Senior pictures, Graduation, Engagement, Musical or Sports events and more
IndySkyPhoto@gmail.com

Facebook: Indy Sky Photo

www.ingramcontent.com/pod-product-compliance
Lightning Source LLC
Chambersburg PA
CBHW061150180526
45170CB00002B/709